A Life
Reclaimed

A Life Reclaimed

How A Quadruple Amputee Regained Control Of Her Life

Sheila May A. Advento

As told to Cynthia Angeles

Dedication

To my family and loved ones; and to the medical, nursing and ancillary staff of the Hackensack University Medical Center and the Kessler Institute for Rehabilitation in Saddle Brook, New Jersey

~ Sheila May A. Advento

Regret

A life of many paths, at times, seem quite meaningless

For we venture into the most superficial,

But, ironically, we shine over.
Materialistic views

Oh how we see of tremendous importance.

But another soul we forget is more important.
Here, underneath my very eyes

A sun hovering over

Bringing me light.

For every waking hour I cherish each passing moment.

I refuse to be the one with any regrets.

~ Sheila May A. Advento

contents

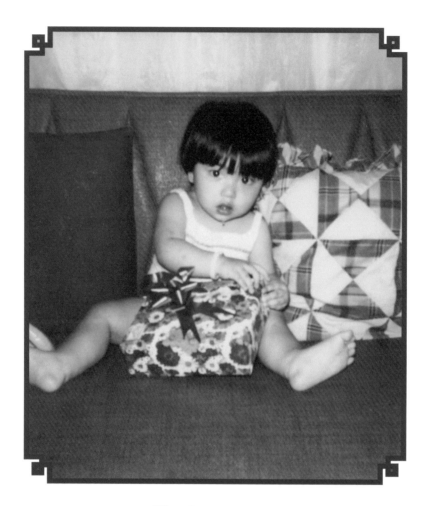

Sheila at age 1

Introduction

Sheila is the youngest of my sister Piedad's three daughters and the youngest of all my nieces and nephews. When she was a little girl in the Philippines, everyone doted on her, especially my late brother Chito, who had five boys. With her light skin, almond eyes, and jet-black hair, she looked like a little Japanese doll that smiled and danced on cue. And how she loved to dance!

Sheila's family migrated to the United States when she was eleven years old. She did very well in school, but seemed to take her time growing up. She loved playing outdoor games with friends and played with her stuffed toys and dolls when she was by herself. To this day, she still hesitates to part with these toys which fill her bedroom. At thirty-two, Sheila is still a child at heart.

Her teenage years were troubled, normal by the standards of her generation, but nonetheless, upsetting to her loved ones. Her decision to drop out of high school in her last year disappointed her family. Yet, through all these years of turmoil, she wrote soulful poems many of which were

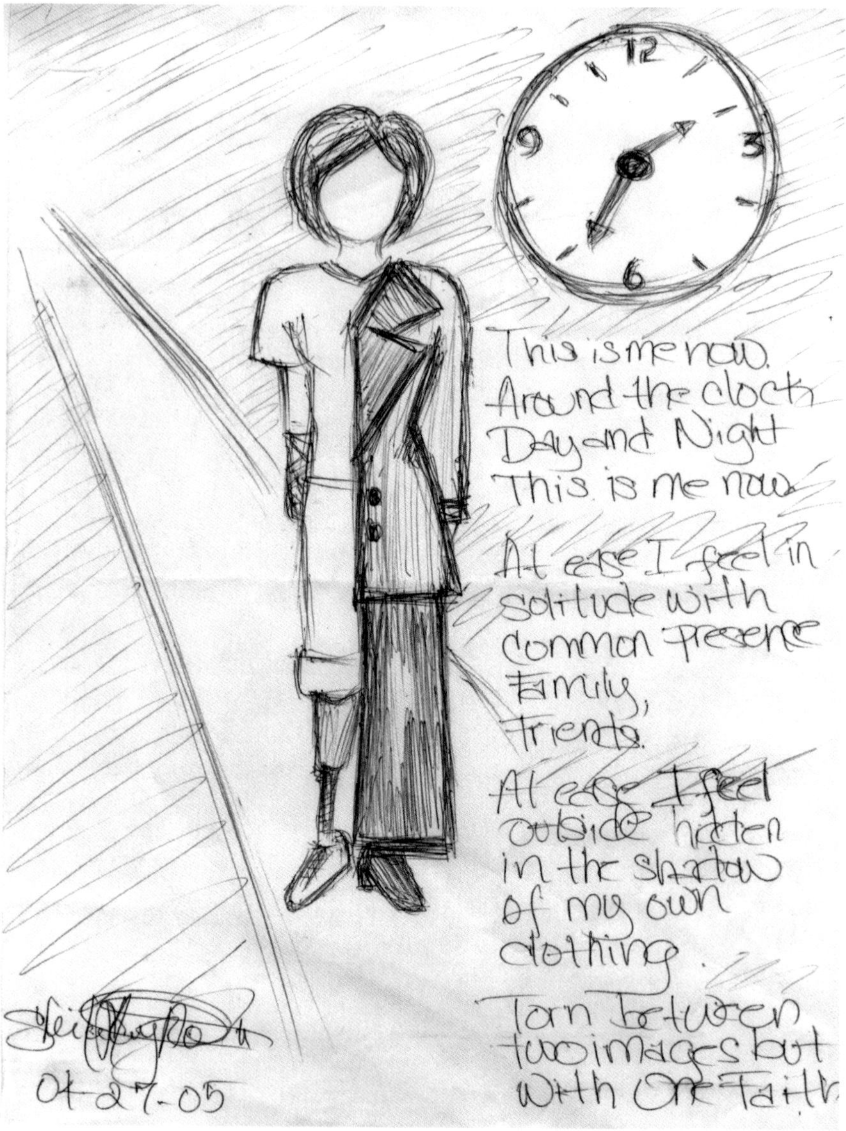
12
9
3
6
This is me now.
Around the clock
Day and Night
This is me now
At ease I feel in
solitude with
common presence
Family,
Friends.
At ease I feel
outside hidden
in the shadow
of my own
clothing.
Torn between
two images but
with One Faith
04-27-05

"The Clock"

published on the internet. She also started working full-time at eighteen, landing various jobs. We only hoped that, one day, she would realize the importance of education and continue her studies.

At nineteen, without telling anyone, Sheila studied for her General Educational Development (GED) credentials, took the test and passed it. Soon thereafter, she found a job at a limousine-leasing firm, and was promoted to supervisor within a few years. She paid her bills dutifully and helped her mom with house expenses. As soon as she was financially able, she attended the Bergen Community College, taking two to three evening courses at a time. She actually enjoyed being back in school and made the Dean's list despite working full time.

Just after she turned twenty-six, Sheila was hired at Quest Diagnostics to work at the Billing/Patient Phone Services Department. Things were certainly looking up for her until tragedy struck. Sheila will tell you what happened.

~Cynthia Angeles, Washington, DC

One: Prelude to Tragedy

Thursday, July 3, 2003:

I went to a bar with some friends. There was much for me to celebrate. I liked working at Quest Diagnostics and enjoyed my night classes at the Bergen Community College. Although I still lived with my mother to save on rent, I helped her a bit by buying groceries periodically and paying the telephone bills. At twenty-six, I was finally on the way to getting my life together.

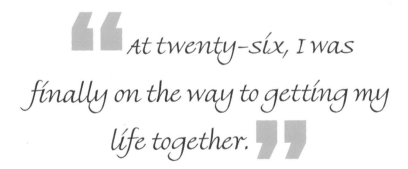

"At twenty-six, I was finally on the way to getting my life together."

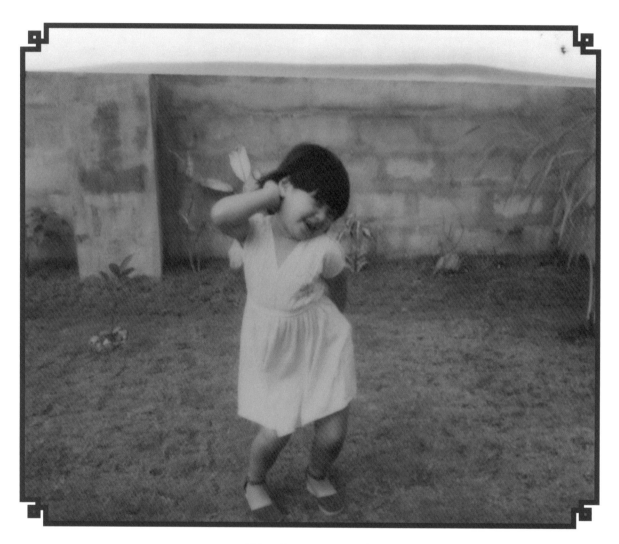

Sheila at age 4

Friday, July 4, 2003:

I was feeling under the weather so my boyfriend at the time, Don, and I stayed indoors and watched television. The following day, Saturday, my sisters, Marsha and Pamela, came with their families to my mother's house for dinner. Don and I joined them but not for too long. I felt weak and had a low-grade fever. I assumed I was coming down with the flu. Hadrien, Pamela's husband, thought it was odd to develop the flu at that time of the year. I took cold/flu tablets which afforded some relief. My symptoms were on and off so no one thought anymore of it—nothing that a good bed rest wouldn't cure.

"There was much for me to celebrate."

Two: Meningococcemia

Sunday, July 6, 2003:

My body rapidly deteriorated. I developed nausea, vomiting, and diarrhea. I had a plastic bag near my bed but kept running in and out of the bathroom. Later, I could no longer stand on my own and saw only shadows on the television screen. My mother, a nurse manager at the New York University Medical Center, came down to the basement to check on me. I complained to her about my difficulty of breathing and blurred vision. She thought I had a viral infection. It was dark in the basement so she turned on the lights to help me see better. Neither of us realized the gravity of my condition at that time.

I crawled back into bed, hoping that the symptoms would pass and that I would feel better in the morning. Not long after, Don called out to my mother for help. I had collapsed on the bathroom floor. She found me gasping for air, unable to move or see, and worse, my lips and fingertips had started to turn purplish-blue. She and Don rushed me to the

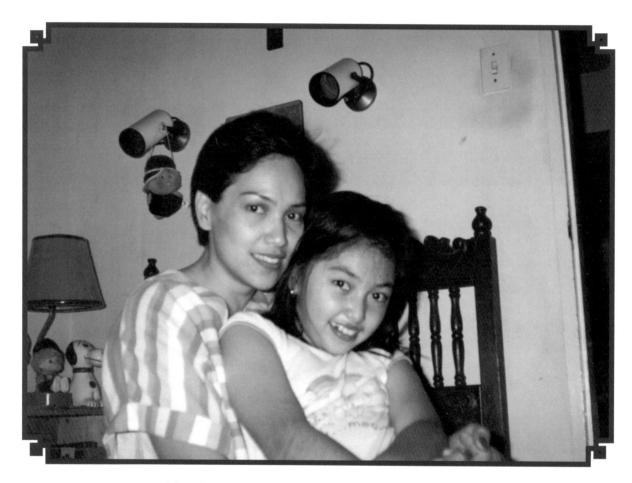

Sheila at age 6 with her mom Piedad

emergency room of Hackensack University Medical Center and alerted everyone in the family.

I was breathing laboriously when we arrived at the hospital. Doctors immediately suspected an infectious disease. With developing fever and dropping blood pressure, I was given three intravenous infusions of broad-spectrum antibiotics. Because my oxygen level was in steep decline, I was hooked to the respirator, but not before getting a heavy dose of sedatives to stop me from resisting intubation. My body organs had shut down in response to the massive infection. My life was slipping away.

> *My life was slipping away.*

Marsha called my father Paquito, and stepmother Jane, who were attending a Christian Life Program (CLP) conference in Seattle. Don waited with my family in the hospital for news of my condition.

Within twenty-four hours, the doctors came up with a definite diagnosis of *meningococcemia*, an acute and potentially life-threatening infection of the bloodstream that commonly leads to *vasculitis* (inflammation of the blood vessels). This disease is caused by airborne bacteria called *Neisseria meningitidis*. This microorganism

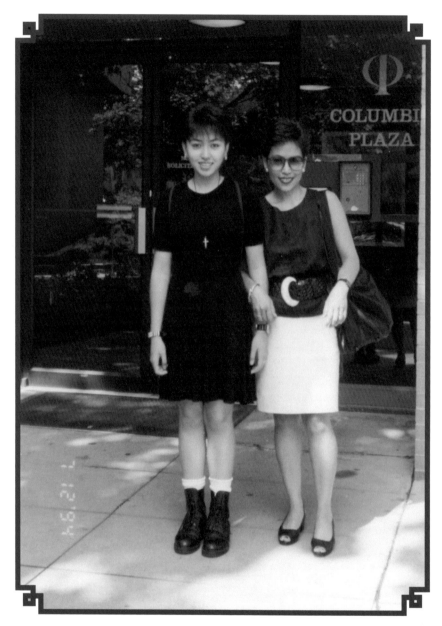

Sheila at 17 with her Tita Cynthia

is acquired by coming into contact with drinking glasses, plates, and utensils used by an infected person, or by breathing in air that was coughed out by infected people. One can easily inhale it from an infected person's breath. I still have no idea where and how I caught it.

> *One can easily inhale it from an infected person's breath.*

Three: A Brush with Death

July 7—14, 2003:

For eight days, I was in a coma in the intensive care unit. My hands and feet had turned dark purple due to insufficient blood supply. Blood had to be diverted to my major organs to revive them. My Catholic family kept vigil and prayed as the days and nights passed with no improvement in my vital signs. Tita Sally ("tita" is the Filipino term for aunt) in the Philippines requested her parish priest to offer Holy Mass, recited *novenas* (nine-day prayers), and even sought the help of a faith healer for my recovery. The news of my illness had reached friends and extended family members who all offered prayers for me. Tita Cynthia, my mother's oldest sister, arrived from Washington, DC. My mother felt my presence in the house every night. Piah, my cousin in California, also sensed my presence in her apartment and heard me crying. "Go back, Sheila, go back," both my mom and my cousin prodded, as if they were imploring my wandering spirit to rejoin my ailing body.

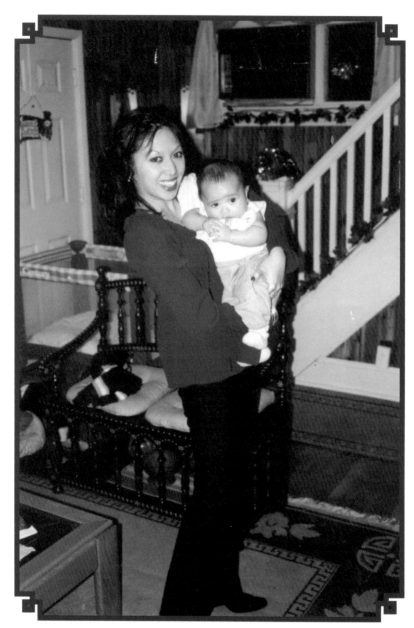

Sheila at 21 with her nephew Justin

My brother-in-law, Hadrien, had a long-time interest in Native American culture and spirituality. He and my sister Pamela studied and lived in New Mexico for several years. There they met Chief Phillip Crazy Bull, a Sicangu Lakota Holy Man from Rosebud, South Dakota. For thirteen years, Hadrien trained with him, and became his "adopted son." In my hospital room, he set up a healing altar (which included a buffalo skull) and conducted healing ceremonies. The Lakota consider the bear as a curing animal. Because of these rituals, I now carry bear spirit and a bear name (*Mato Suksuta Win*, meaning Hard Bear Woman).

During my long period of unconsciousness, Chief Crazy Bull led a Sun Dance ceremony—a Native American ceremony which represents life and rebirth of all living things. In this ceremony, hundreds of people dance, fast, and pray for days. On the fourth day, the Sun Dancers are pierced in the chest and tied there by ropes, which are attached to the upper part of the Sacred Tree (usually a cottonwood tree). Piercing is the most sacred part of this ceremony and symbolizes the personal sacrifice that the participant makes for the welfare of the tribe or for special favors to benefit others. Chief Crazy Bull and the other Sun Dancers made the sacrifice so that I may live. He came to visit us a few months later and conducted an *inipi* (sweat

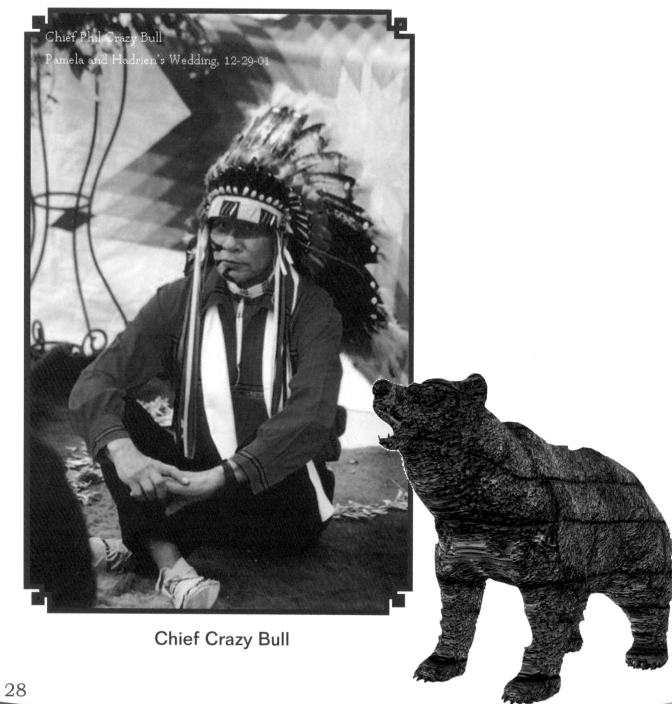

Chief Phil Crazy Bull
Pamela and Hadrien's Wedding, 12-29-01

Chief Crazy Bull

lodge) ceremony which I attended. It is a Native American healing ceremony for the purification of mind, body, spirit, and heart. That was the last time I saw him.

He died on January 18, 2006 of a heart attack.

"Because of these rituals, I now carry bear spirit and a bear name (Mato Suksuta Win, meaning Hard Bear Woman)."

Four: where am I?

Monday, July 14, 2003:

On day eight, the intensivist (critical care doctor) and the nursing staff called my family to a conference to discuss my medical status. The doctor basically said that his team had done the best they could to reverse my condition, with no positive results, and hinted that perhaps, it was time to terminate the treatments. My family convened and refused to give up on me. They felt strongly and fervently hoped that I would pull through. At that time, my mother was the only one in the family who really understood the medical details. She suggested to the intensivist not to stop supportive treatments, but that I be weaned off intravenous sedation. She also said that if my vital signs continued to deteriorate, then no extreme measures should be attempted. That day, the prospect of having to pull the plug hovered over all of them like a dark, threatening cloud.

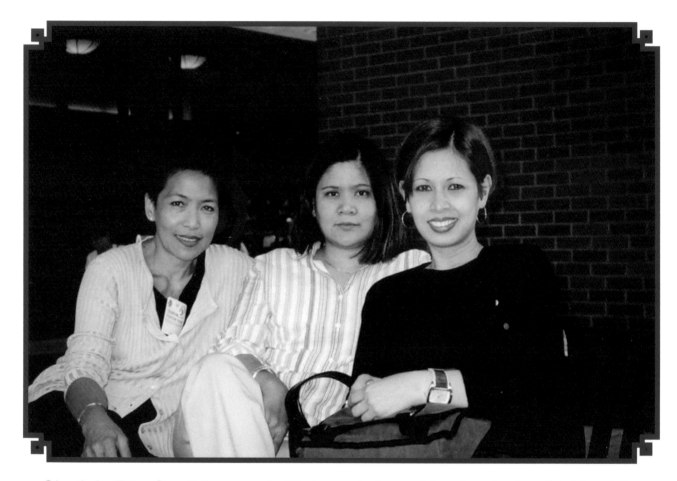

Sheila's Tita Cynthia, cousin Piah, and sister Marsha during Piah's visit at the Hackensack University Medical Center in July 2003

Tuesday, July 15, 2003:

I opened my eyes on the morning of day nine. Pamela walked into my room and took her usual seat next to my bed. When she saw my open eyes, she was shocked. I tried to speak, but could not because of the tube inserted in my throat. The nursing staff and my family were alerted. When I was able to speak, though barely understandable, I told Pamela about my long and exhausting trip to Calcutta, India. There I found myself wandering around in an open market. It was very bright, yet so empty, and there was music. As the volume got louder and louder, I got scared and started running. Then I met my late maternal grandmother who gently urged me to return home. I think I did — when I finally woke up.

> *My whole family was tearful but jubilant to have me back.*

My whole family was tearful but jubilant to have me back. The following day, Piah, who had flown in from California, came to visit me. It was wonderful to see her and the rest of

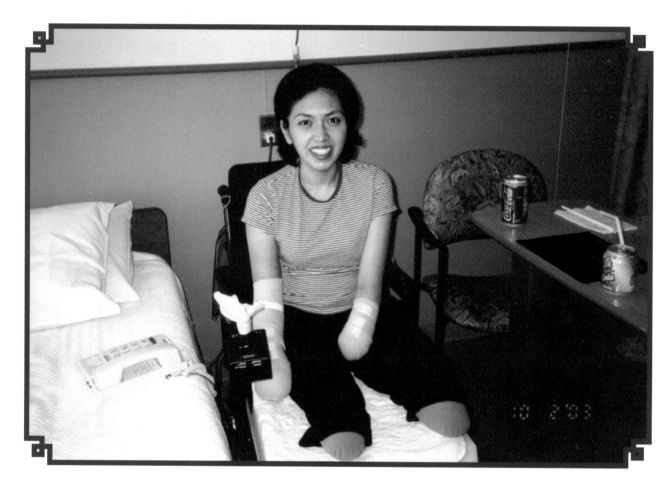

Sheila at Kessler Institute for Rehabilitation

my family. Indeed, it felt great to be alive, but I knew there were problems.

My mother, anticipating my needs, requested psychiatric evaluation. Despite my initial protest, I was given an anti-depressant which I took until the day I finally went home. The other priority was to regain my strength so I ate as much as I could. Most importantly, a major decision had to be made. My hands and feet had turned almost black and lifeless and might have to be amputated. My intensivist suggested hyperbaric treatment, which meant putting me in a chamber of pure oxygen, hoping that it would bring life back to my limbs.

I stayed inside the chamber, a clear tube, for fourteen sessions, and lay still for two hours each day. On my first treatment, Pamela accompanied me. The chamber looked weird and terrifying. After being locked in for fifteen minutes, I panicked and screamed to her to let me out. I felt relieved when we returned to my room but I knew I had to try it again, and I did. Days passed and eventually, I completed the required treatments. We were so thrilled because the color of my limbs went almost back to normal. We all thought the treatment had worked. I even tried walking with the therapists, but it became too painful to take even a few

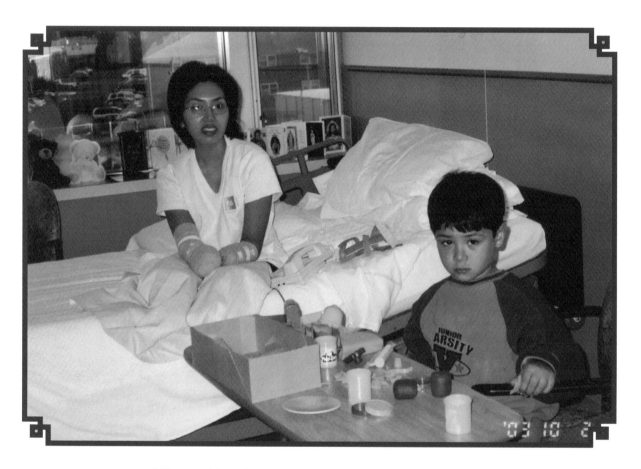

Albert (Albi) visiting with his Aunt Sheila

steps. I had visions of my family taking turns in carrying me everywhere and I knew that would not work. A few days later, I developed a fever—a sign of infection that had to be dealt with.

Five: To Live or Not

My mom and I discussed the choice we had to make—amputate or probably die from the infection. There was no question that I wanted to live. I had felt from the start that my limbs had to go and that the hyperbaric treatment would be a waste of time. Without hesitation, I told her, "Cut them off! Let's just get this over with!" I had no idea what challenges lay ahead.

From the ICU, I was transferred to a big, cheery, private room with a plasma TV on the eighth floor. Aware of what was about to happen, I cried uncontrollably. I felt depressed and lost. Only the constant presence of my family and friends, day and night, kept me strong to face my ordeal. They were in my room tending to my needs, chatting, eating, joking, having fun, helping me carry my burden one day at a time. I did not eat much, but when I did, I shunned hospital food. Everybody brought food, especially Jane, who cooked special dishes for me and the others. In August and September 2003, I went through multiple surgeries.

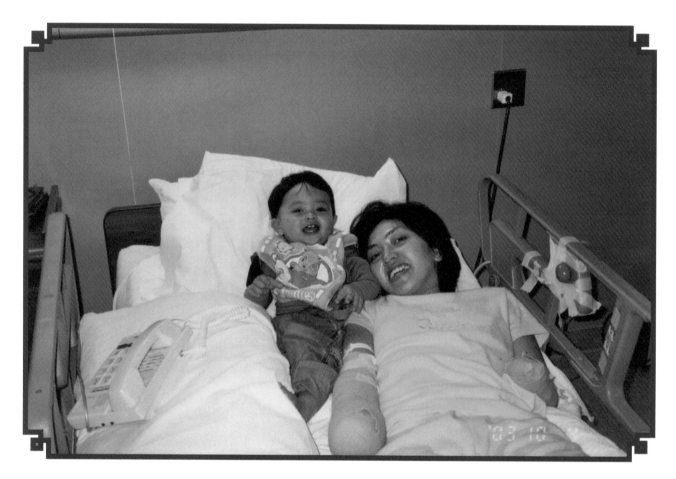

Sheila with nephew Justin

Wednesday, August 13, 2003:

The first was the amputation of my arms (below the elbows). I had not been warned that they would do the surgery that particular day. I was undergoing another procedure so the surgeon decided to do the amputation at the same time. When I woke up, I still had a phantom feeling in my hands. The moment I realized they had been cut off, I felt so distressed and traumatized. I could not stop crying and all my family could do was to comfort me.

" There was no question that I wanted to live. "

Monday, August 18, 2003:

The second surgery was the amputation of my legs (below the knees). This was unbearably painful so I was given pain killers intravenously, and by mouth. At that point, I felt physically different, but with all four limbs amputated, who wouldn't? I felt helpless and disheartened, all the time thinking I was no longer whole. "What could I possibly accomplish now? Will I still have a social life? Who

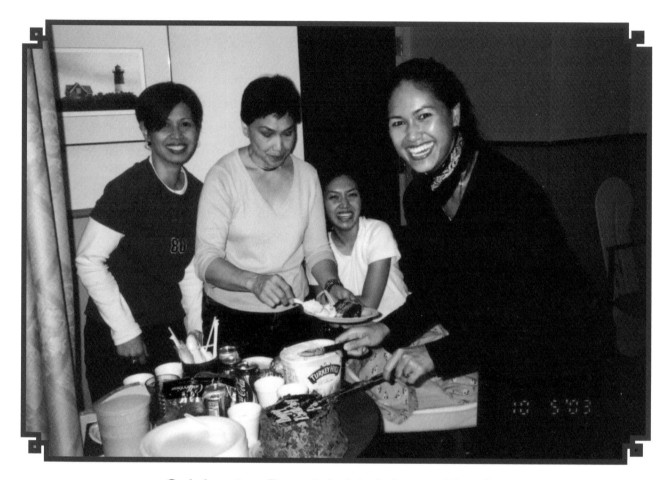

Celebrating Pamela's birthday at Kessler
From left: Marsha, Piedad, Sheila, Pamela

would want me now?!" Indeed, only my family's constant presence and support gave me courage to go on. I knew they would not abandon me. My dad even said that, if necessary, he would quit his job to take care of me. And, no matter what, my mother was always there for us.

Because they did not want to leave me alone at all, my mom or someone else would stay the night in my room. Tita Cynthia came from Washington, DC, very often to keep me company and give my parents some respite. The nursing staff understood and accommodated our needs. I had a chair that converted into a bed and they provided us with extra towels, pillows, sheets, and blankets.

> " *My dad even said that, if necessary, he would quit his job to take care of me.* "

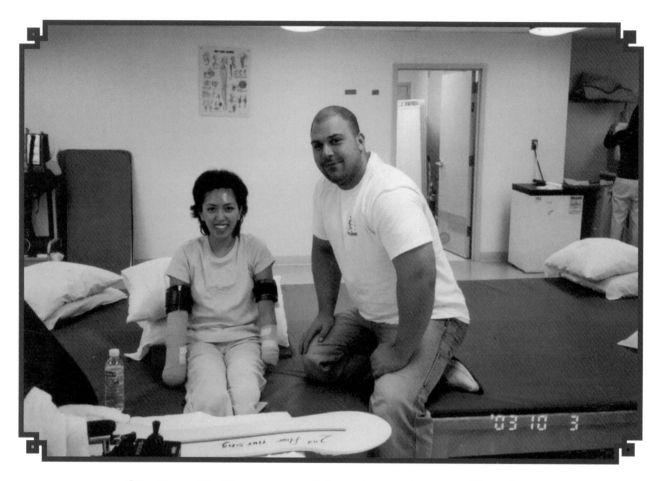

Sheila with Dan, one of her therapists at Kessler

September 10, 2003:

For my third surgery, a piece of muscle taken from my back and skin from my left thigh were grafted to my right arm in preparation for a possible hand transplant in the future. This is the reason why my right arm is longer than my left. The surgery lasted ten long hours. With all the patch-up work done on me, I must have looked like a broken Raggedy Ann doll.

While I was in post-op, my family was extra-vigilant about my condition. My mother made sure I was given the proper care. Because the hospital staff knew she was a nurse manager at the Rusk Institute of Rehabilitation Medicine at the NYU Medical Center, they listened to her and respected her input.

Once I was back in my regular room, my family relaxed. I started regaining my strength although I still did not eat much. I had many visitors besides my mother, father, and Jane; most came even before I had the surgeries. When Rose, a friend whom I had not seen in six years, showed up, I was overwhelmed. Abie, another friend who had moved to Florida, also came with her family. My cousin Norman's wife, Minnie, a flight attendant based in Hong Kong, also took time from her brief layover in New York to see me. My father's and stepmother's colleagues at the Christian Life Program

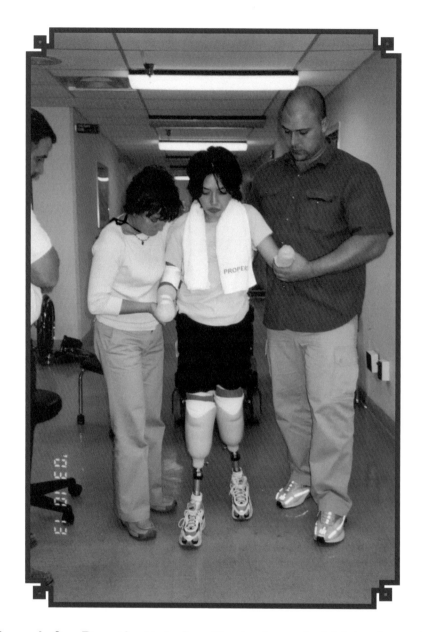

From left: Prosthetist Joe Reda (partly hidden), and
flanking Sheila, her therapists, Eva and Dan

visited and prayed for my recovery. Marsha, Pamela, and Hadrien were permanent fixtures at the hospital. Marsha's husband at the time, Albert, brought my nephews, Albi and Justin, to cheer me up. My father dropped by during his lunch break and visited after work. His good sense of humor helped lighten up the mood in the room. Jocelyn, a close family friend, joined the crowd as often as she could. Lenny, my mother's boyfriend (now my stepfather) visited many times and was as concerned about me as he was about my mother. My personal assistant, Eve, was very warm and caring. A strong woman from Zimbabwe, she carried me from my bed to a chair and back without any problems or complaints. She also made me laugh.

> *Once I was back in my regular room, my family relaxed.*

My room was filled with food, flowers, cards, and stuffed toys, including a Raggedy Ann doll which Marsha bought for me. The hospital staff often said that it didn't feel like a hospital in my room. It was comforting to have family and friends around everyday.

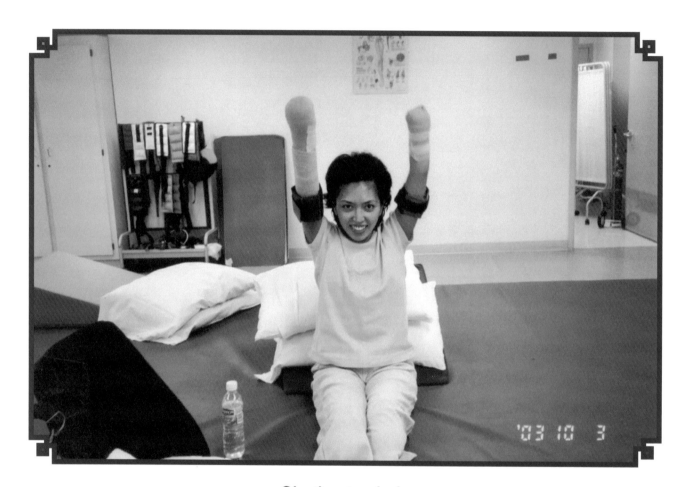

Sheila at rehab

They helped me a lot. God blessed me with loving people. Even the nurses were very kind. One of them, Laura, even brought her sisters to the hospital one day to pamper me with beauty treatments (shampoo, blow-dry, waxing). The thoughtful gesture warmed my heart and the treatments really gave me a much-needed lift.

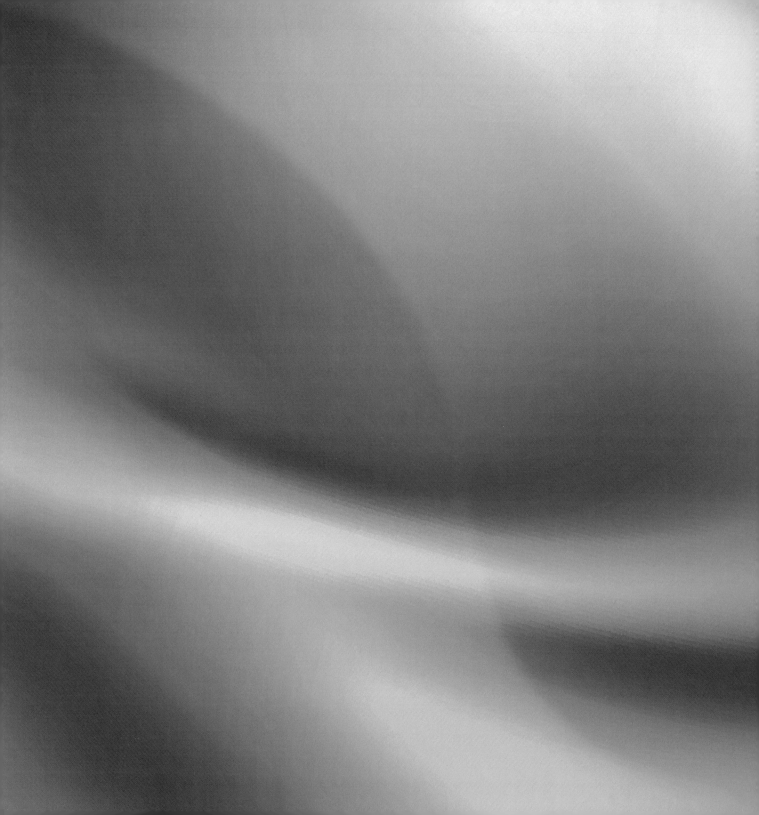

Six: To Walk Again—With Prosthetics

Tuesday, September 30, 2003:

I finally left Hackensack University Medical Center and was transferred to the Kessler Institute for Rehabilitation in Saddle Brook, New Jersey. For one month, I went through extensive therapy: two sessions a day (occupational and physical), five to six days a week. Crunches, leg exercises, arm work-outs—I did them all. I was bed-ridden for two months in the hospital, so my exercise regime was challenging. I started eating more, not only because I was more active, but because I really liked the food there.

I remember getting my pair of prosthetic legs. When I first saw them, I could not imagine how I could stand with them. The top were molds for my legs connected to the feet by metal rods. Eve, Jane and Jocelyn were around when I first tried them on. It was tough but I practiced everyday—getting up from a sitting position and walking; at first with a walker, and later on, while my therapists held on to me. I worked

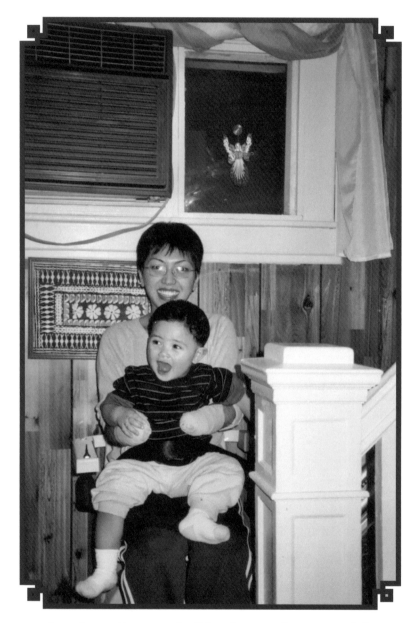

Justin riding with Sheila on the stair lift

so hard that I bonded with my therapists including John, Michael, Eva, and Dan, and my prosthetist, Joe Reda. Joe walked around with his tools stashed in his pockets. He would watch me during my sessions, pull out his tools and start making adjustments on my prostheses.

When I finally walked around the gym by myself with John and Dan watching and following behind me, I felt victorious. I cried with joy! Dan said that he had to look away or he would break down and cry along with me. The other patients in therapy applauded. My dad witnessed me walk from my room to the hallway for the first time. Then, I surprised my mom when she walked out of the elevator and saw me walking in the hallway. Yes, I was like a baby taking its first steps, but I felt ever so proud. And so did my parents!

Seven: Coming Home

Thursday, October 30, 2003:

> *Yes, I was like a baby taking its first steps, but I felt ever so proud.*

I was released from Kessler. Going home was very exciting. I had waited so long for that moment. My mother had a stair lift installed to get me to and from my temporary bedroom on the second floor of the house. My little nephew Justin enjoyed "riding" up and down the stairs with me.

Being home was heartwarming but it exposed all my physical challenges. I used a manual wheelchair to get me from my bedroom to the bathroom and back. Mommy or Eve carried me from the wheelchair to the toilet or bath bench for my showers. Independent as I was before my illness, not being able to perform these basic tasks frustrated and angered me. Despite all these difficulties, I never asked, "Why did this happen to me?" I realized everything happened for a

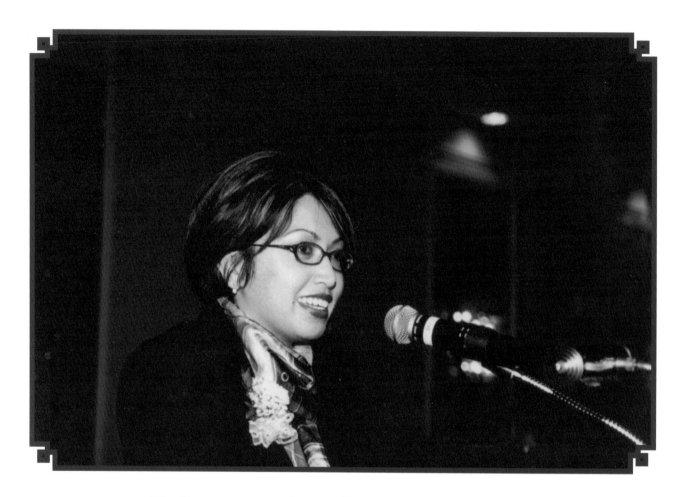

**Sheila speaking during Kessler's William Kingman
Page Memorial Alumni Award ceremonies in
December 2004**

reason and felt so lucky to be alive.

For a while, I received home therapy, which included a kit of adaptive equipment and devices to enable me to eat, use the toilet, clean myself, etc. A couple of therapists worked with me until I was able to go back to Kessler as an outpatient for occupational therapy. There, I was taught many tips on how to survive without limbs. I felt safe in rehab and did not absorb much of what was being taught. I just laughed and smiled my way through the sessions most of the time. But once it was over, I realized how difficult life was outside my safety zone. I have always been someone who took things in stride. I would keep going despite any upsets in my life or merely laugh them off. This time, it caught up with me.

Because of my pride and stubborn streak, I chose not to get psychiatric counseling and refused to take any anti-depressants. I guess I wanted to try surviving without professional help or pills. Besides, I took too many pills at the hospital and at Kessler and didn't want to be dependent on them. Thankfully, my mother was always around to explain and validate the emotions I was going through. She often posed this question to me: "Imagine being alone in the desert or an island. What would you do to survive?"

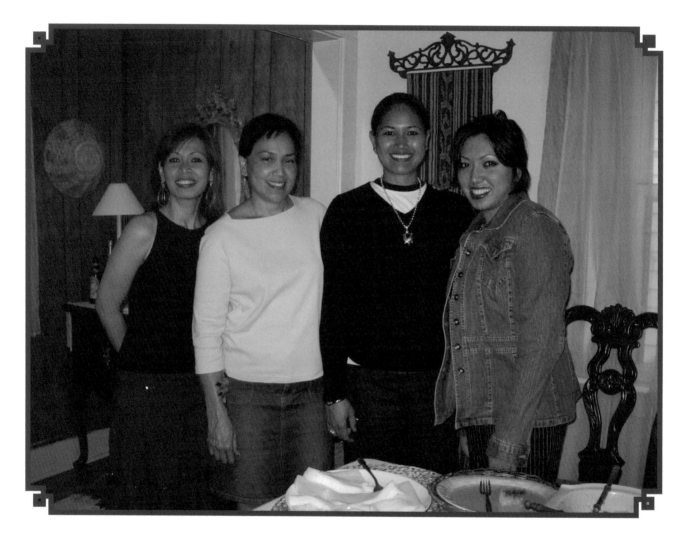

From left: Marsha, Piedad, Pamela, and Sheila, during
Pam's birthday/baby shower in October 2005

Then she would say, "Use whatever is left of you to survive. Crawl if you have to. Use your stump to eat if need be." My mom was tough with me. When I was in the hospital, she instructed me to keep track of my medication. "Doctors and nurses are human beings. They make mistakes, too. It is up to you to manage your care." Sometimes, I would accuse her of treating me like a patient, not her daughter. I thought she was too harsh with me. Despite my angry outbursts, I listened hard. Now I realize that without her tough love and encouragement, I wouldn't have progressed as much as I have. She instilled in me the importance of learning to adapt to my physical challenges in order to reclaim my life.

Eight: My Prosthetic Hands

Sometime in March 2004, I received my body-powered prosthetic hands. Simply put, it is a contraption that is strapped on my shoulders with the hand prosthetics at the end. It is rather heavy and bulky. In hot weather, it can be uncomfortable. I usually wear a short-sleeved T-shirt underneath to avoid chafing my upper arms and cover the whole thing up with a long-sleeved shirt when I go out. It took me a while to get used to it. To eat, a fork or spoon is inserted into an eating brace which I grip with my "right hand." Of course, I need someone to slice my food into bite-sized pieces. And I use a straw to drink.

> *My mom was tough with me.*

Needless to say, I went through many emotional roller-coasters along the way. I would get frustrated with my condition, get angry and cry, but my mother would assure me that it was all right to cry. I always had high expectations of myself but was

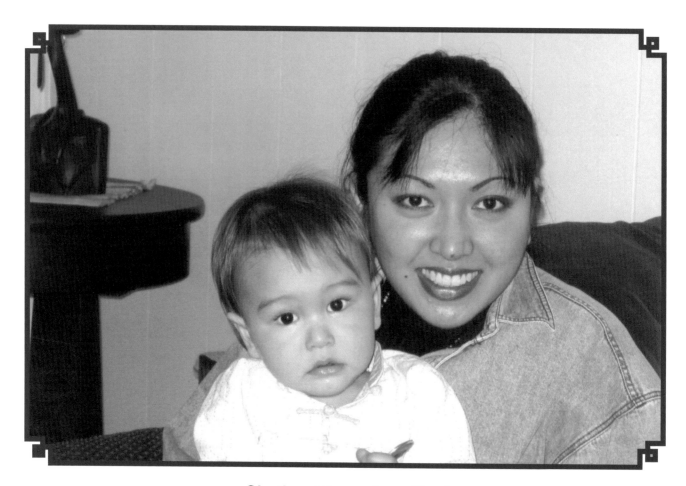

Sheila with nephew Paolo

not quite prepared to face the challenges of daily living as a quadruple amputee. Everyday was a learning experience and thanks to the patience, understanding, and support of my family, I made a lot of progress.

Eventually, I moved to the basement which was slightly modified to accommodate my needs. Because I didn't use a wheel chair, there was no need for a ramp. There is a side door which I could use but rarely did. Instead, I learned how to go up and down the stairs which led to the kitchen and out the backdoor. The steps leading to the backyard were also widened for my easy access.

One of my surgeons thought that I would be more "functional" with a pair of myoelectric hand prostheses. However, my insurance would only cover the body-powered hand prosthetics. In desperation, Tita Cynthia wrote a letter of plea to Dr. Harold Sears, president and general manager of Motion Control, a Utah-based company which makes myoelectric arm prostheses. In response, Dr. Sears kindly arranged for a loaner through Joe Reda. I requested the left arm because my right arm was a bit longer than the left and I was afraid there would be complications with the fittings. Sadly, it was a continuous struggle to use the left myoelectric arm because I am right-handed. Moreover, the

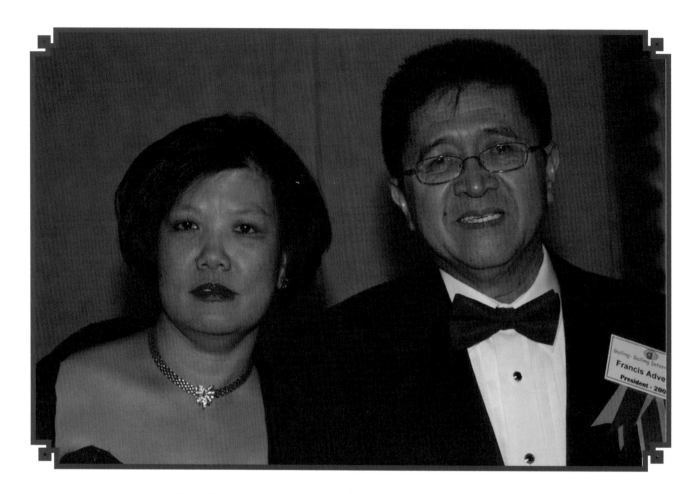

Sheila's stepmother Jane and father Paquito

myoelectric hand would sometimes malfunction. The fingers would open and close continuously without intervention on my part. In the end, I returned the loaner because I simply could not cope with it. I stuck with my body-powered prosthetic hands to which I have adjusted nicely. Nevertheless, my family and I will always be grateful to Dr. Sears for providing me with such rare opportunity. Although he warned us that myoelectric arms are not for everyone, he also stressed the importance of adequate occupational therapy for it to work. Perhaps, myoelectric arms are not for me.

"Needless to say, I went through many emotional roller-coasters along the way."

Nine: Inspiration

In December 2004, I was named one of the recipients of the William Kingman Page Memorial Alumni Award for Kessler Institute for Rehabilitation, for outstanding achievement during rehabilitation. I was also featured in Kessler's 2006 calendar (I was April), along with fellow survivors.

One of the aides at Kessler, Rudy Delgado, who became a dear friend, asked if he could take photos of me while undergoing rehabilitation, for a school project. I agreed and eventually collaborated with him to create a pictorial book entitled *Inspiration*. It features black-and-white photographs of me during my month of therapy at Kessler and incorporates snippets of my experience, my drawings, and poems, all written with my prosthetic hand. This book was never developed for publication.

A Life Reclaimed is not intended to replicate *Inspiration*. It is simply my way of telling my story—a story of survival, acceptance, and courage to live. It is also about my continuing struggle as a quadruple amputee, to achieve as much

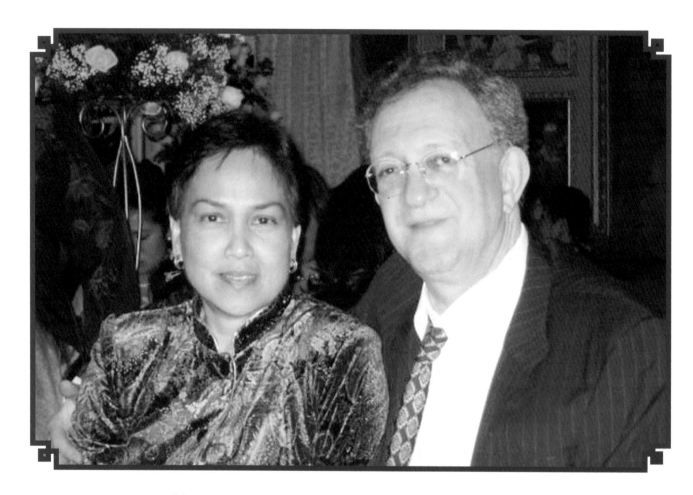

Sheila's mother Piedad and stepfather Lenny

normalcy in my life as I can and to regain more control over it. I hope that you will share it with someone you know or love.

> " *I hope that you will share it with someone you know or love.* "

Epilogue

I truly believe one's level of recovery is up to one's mental and emotional strength. Vanity, in good measure, can be a motivating factor.

I have always been very careful with my appearance. I often shopped for clothes and shoes, and changed hairstyles frequently. I went to beauty salons for manicures and pedicures occasionally but did my nails myself most of the time. I loved red nail polish, but tried other colors, too. In the emergency room, it upset me when the nurse removed the polish on one finger nail. It was the purple one that Marsha gave me.

With my prosthetics, I don't have to worry about painting my nails anymore, but I see no reason to stop caring about my appearance despite my limitations. I wash and style my own hair when it is short. When it is long, I need help to comb and put it up. I learned how to apply my makeup with, first, my prosthetic hand, then, with my stump. Someone has to set up everything in front of me, though. Getting dressed is a lot easier and faster with somebody's help, but I have done

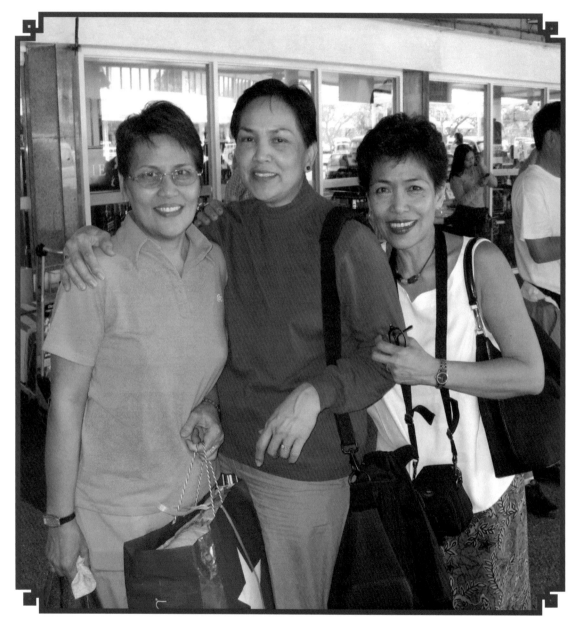

Sheila's Tita Sally, mother Piedad, and Tita Cynthia in Manila in 2007

it myself quite a few times. I still wear jewelry (except rings for obvious reasons) and keep a selection of sneakers, boots, and dressy shoes to match my outfits.

Losing my limbs was a huge challenge to my physical, mental, and emotional well-being. Imagine having to learn how to sit, stand, walk, and touch again—just like a baby, but, this time, with the prosthetics. Coming home after a month of therapy and rehabilitation at Kessler, I was enveloped by the warmth and love of my family and friends. Fearful of what was out there, conscious and scared of people staring at my prostheses, I avoided going out. When I had to, I wore big, long-sleeved shirts and roomy trousers to accommodate and cover my hand and leg prostheses. But after a year of recuperation, I couldn't bear being sheltered anymore. The reality of what I used to be (pretty wild, my mom would say) kept pushing me to get on with my life. Gradually, I reintroduced myself to a social life. I began to go out with my old friends and met new ones. Through my father and stepmother, I joined the Christian Life Program where I was able to speak about my experiences to large audiences on numerous occasions.

I even dated again! It hasn't been easy, but coming to terms with being a quadruple amputee, rather than dwelling on it, somehow made it more manageable. I remember going to a

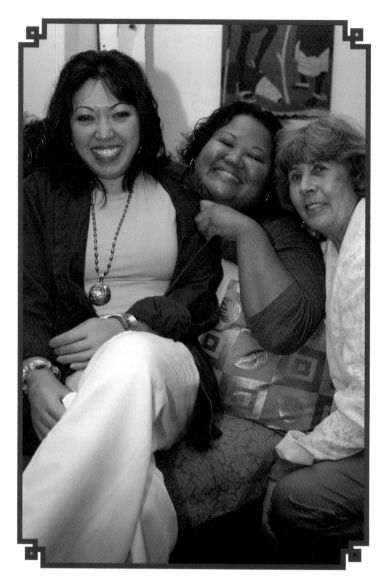

Sheila and her friends Abie and Carol

restaurant-bar in Ridgewood with Rose. Her brother Chuck was there with his friends who did not know about my prosthetics. One guy came over and introduced himself to us. When he shook my hand, he was so shocked he blurted out, "Whoa!" I laughed so hard we all ended up laughing.

Because there was so much I did before that I could no longer do, I have learned to be creative. To write or draw, I have someone wrap rubber bands around my pens and pencils so my prosthetic hand can easily grip them. My penmanship has not suffered, thankfully, and my drawings are not too bad, either. I can also send text messages pretty well with my stump. My cell phone has a speaker phone which is essential.

I've always loved dancing, even as a child, and used to go dancing a lot. I also liked to sing and frequented karaoke clubs with friends. Thank God I am able to dance with my prosthetics! I have gone dancing only a few times, though, including a brave attempt to do the "Electric Slide", which I enjoyed immensely. I have not lost my spirit of adventure either. Last year, I went to Hershey Park and tried the gripping roller coaster and a few other rides. It was great fun! Recently, I felt like jumping and did. Not a high one, mind you, but it felt good to do it!

In July 2004, I went back to work at Quest Diagnostics.

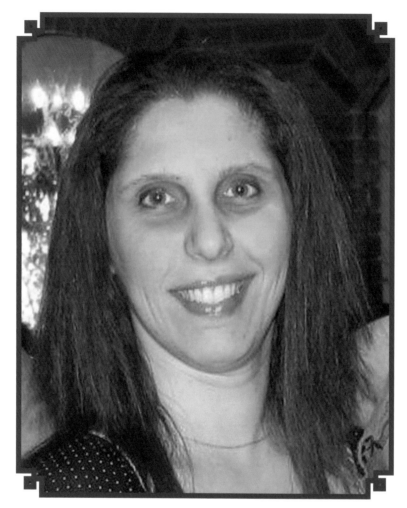

Sheila's friend Rose

The staff and management welcomed me with open arms. They were incredibly supportive of me. Initially, I planned to work only part-time, but, since this option was not available, I decided to try a full-time position. It has been close to five years now and I am still with Quest, albeit part-time. I work in the Medical Billing/Patient Phone Services Department. Like my colleagues, I take calls, assist customers and patients with their bills, and write down insurance details. Many times, I speak to clients (doctors' offices) and insurance companies to get necessary information. There are only a couple of modifications I utilize - typing pegs and a cordless headset in the beginning; I have since switched to the regular headset. I may not be as quick as I was before my illness, but I am fast enough to keep up with the demands of my job.

In July 2005, my co-workers at Quest started a fundraising campaign to help me purchase a pair of myoelectric hands which my insurance would not cover. They printed and sold 1000 raffle tickets at $5 each to donate to the "Helping Hands Fund." They even sold doughnuts, bagels, and coffee everyday in their offices to add to the Fund. The campaign spread outside Quest through my family and friends. The Fund received donations from New York, California, West Virginia, and the Washington, DC area. Unfortunately, the fundraising was discontinued and the amount raised was barely sufficient

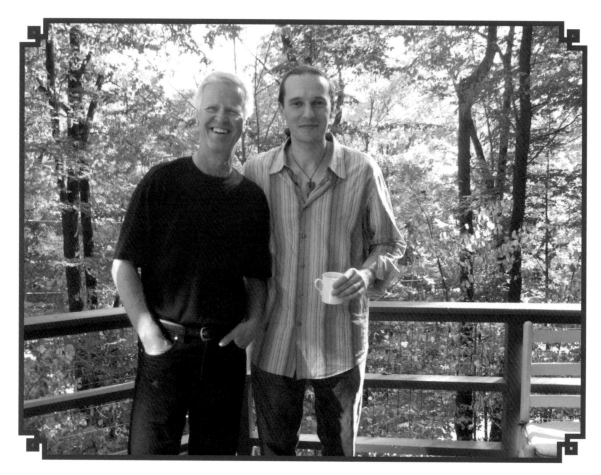

Michael, Cynthia's husband, and
Hadrien, Sheila's brother-in-law
(Pamela's husband)

to purchase one myoelectric arm. In the end, I gave up on the idea of getting one. Through the years, I have become adequately functional with my body-powered hand prostheses and my stumps. Besides, I found the myoelectric hand more difficult to manage and control.

Technology is getting better with time and I am hoping that lighter body-powered hand prostheses will be available in the near future. In the meantime, I will keep forging ahead with what I have.

Being able to type and write with my hand prostheses has enabled me to continue my studies at the Bergen Community College through online courses. Although I have done this off and on in the past several years, I managed to remain on the Dean's list. I would like to continue my studies and pursue an associate degree in broadcast journalism and public speaking. Fortunately, I have been given permission to use the unused funds from the fundraiser to realize this goal.

In September 2005, I ventured on my own. Don, still a friend, helped me move to my first apartment. Recently, I moved to my third place, a cute one-bedroom apartment, also in Hackensack, New Jersey, and about a ten-minute drive to my mother's house. Renting my own place is a financial strain,

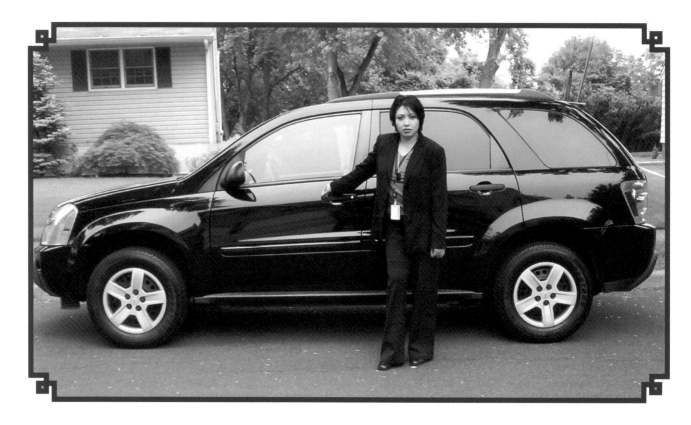

Sheila and her black SUV

but I needed to do it. I enjoy keeping house and stress about responsibilities such as vacuuming the floor, just like everyone else. Somehow, it makes me feel undefeated.

And, I am a driver again. After a lot of time, research, and patience I am back behind the wheel —in a black SUV. It's funny because my driving style hasn't changed. The only difference is that my car is equipped with gadgets such as a hand control for the steering wheel, a button for my left knee to activate the signals, a hand control on the left to control both the gas and the brakes, and a rain sensor so I don't have to manually operate the wipers. For me, driving again was a major leap towards independence. Now, I can go places without having to depend on others. I have even driven to Cold Springs, NY, Pennsylvania, and Washington, DC. More than anything else, driving has given me back some control over my life and a semblance of normalcy as well.

" *And, I am a driver again.* "

Of course, I have my frustrations, too, and still harbor a lot of insecurities. I always worry about the visual effect that my hand prostheses has on people, more so because my right arm is technically longer than

81

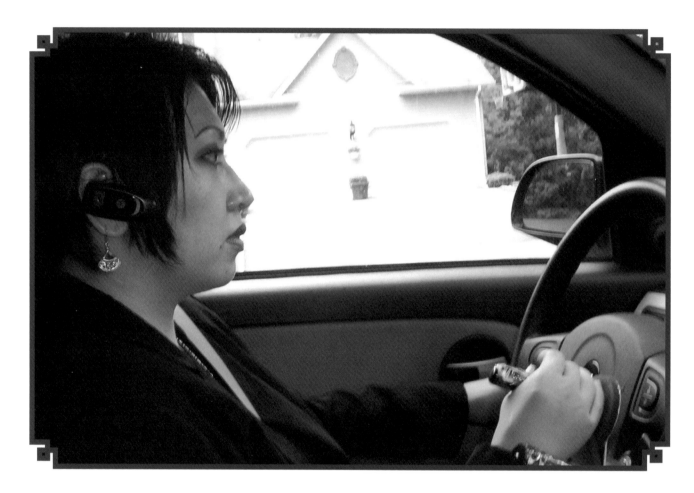

Sheila in her car

my left. I am super conscious when my "hands" get dirty. We have used soap, gasoline, and all kinds of detergents to clean them, but nothing has worked.

When someone who is unaware of my condition is about to shake my hand, I immediately warn that person about my prosthetics. I don't want him or her to get surprised or shocked. So far, no one has shied away from shaking my prosthetic hands.

Obviously, there are limitations to what I can do with my prostheses or even my stumps, so I depend on personal assistants, family, and friends for help. I have had several personal assistants since Eve left. One of them was Lina, a hard-working Filipino mother who went back to her family in the Philippines after living with me and my mother for a year. The other was Carol, who was with me the longest and whom I consider one of my best friends. She has since retired and lives with her daughter and family in Darby, Pennsylvania. Both Lina and Carol were extremely patient and tolerant of my occasional mood swings. It is, after all, a challenge to wake up every morning knowing that I am a quadruple amputee. Nevertheless, I have accomplished much since leaving Kessler Institute for Rehabilitation in October 2003, and I intend to do more.

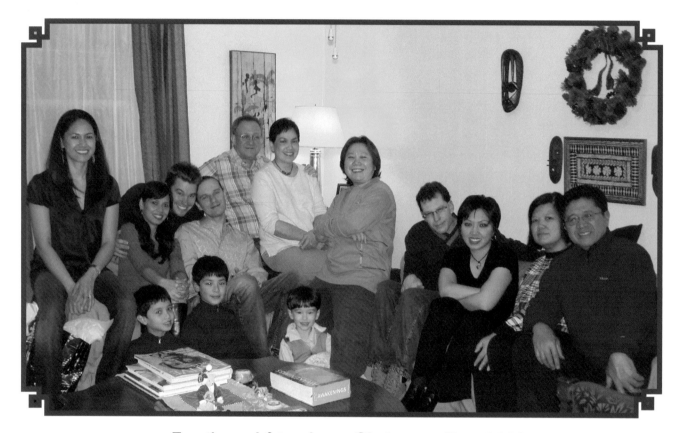

Family and friends on Christmas Day 2008

From left: Pamela, Marsha, Marsha's boyfriend Michael, Hadrien,
Lenny, Piedad, Jocelyn, Joe, Sheila, Jane, and Paquito
Front row: Justin, Albert, and Paolo

> **"***I am a quadruple amputee. Nevertheless, I have accomplished much.***"**

I have had a couple of relationships since my amputations, including a marriage that didn't work out. About two years ago, I met someone who provided me with tremendous moral support at a time when I needed it the most. For this, I am thankful, and I do feel lucky to have been in normal relationships despite my disability.

My parents were divorced in 1992 and are both remarried now. The long road to reconciliation was not an easy one but we have all learned to accept and adjust. In the end, it simply broadened our family network —not divided it. Almost every weekend, sometimes twice a week, we all convene at my mom's house for pot luck lunch or dinner. Lenny takes a break from his books and joins us. He likes most Filipino dishes but won't eat pork (he is Jewish). My dad and Jane live just a block away so they join us most of the time. Jane usually cooks and helps my mom with the washing up. Pam, Hadrien, and their son, Paolo, come all the way from Cold Springs, NY, an hour's drive away. Marsha, her boyfriend, Michael, and the kids, Albert and Justin, are almost always around. We have squabbles and

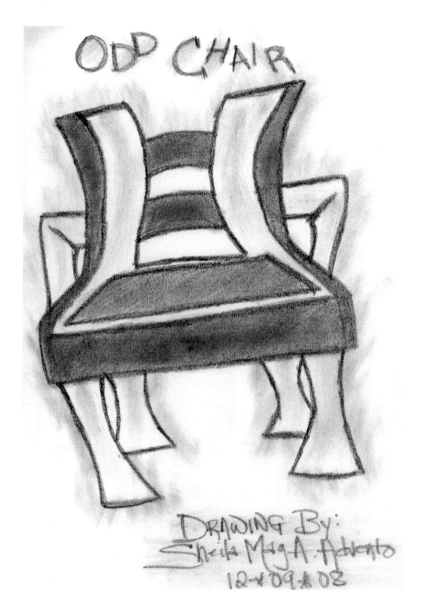

"The Odd Chair"

little quarrels just like a normal family. But we are closely knit and always in touch.

I will always be grateful to each one of them for being there for me at every step of the way. I know I have frustrated, angered, and disappointed them countless times in my life but they were always there when I needed them. I thank my father for his love; Jane for doing her utmost to help; Marsha, her boyfriend Michael, Pamela, and Hadrien for listening and reaching out to me. I cannot thank my mother enough for her tough love and understanding, her iron will to get me the best possible care available, and to keep me focused in rebuilding my life.

I am a quadruple amputee. It has been almost six years since my surgeries and I still have difficulty facing up to this reality. I wake up every day aware of the "tasks" that lie ahead of me: putting on my prosthetic legs and hands, getting ready for work, driving to work, and all the other normal activities of living. I am no longer the independent woman I once was. I have to rely on help now. But these challenges push me to go on. I have fallen many times and somehow managed to get up each time. My family, friends, and associates are all very supportive, and I am so lucky to have them. I must also say that I am fortunate to live in New Jersey's Bergen County. Its Department of Human

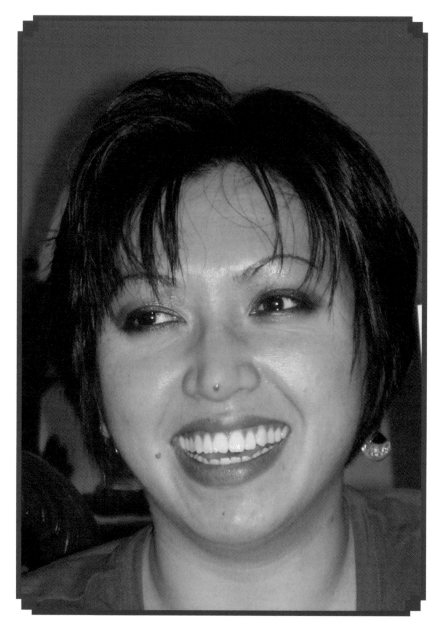

Sheila on her 32nd birthday, April 2009

Services, specifically the Division of Disability Services and the Division of Vocational Rehabilitation, has been very helpful to me ever since I applied for assistance. The support they have extended to me made so much difference in my recovery.

Life has been hard; but life has also been kind. I have been blessed with another chance to make a difference not only to myself, but to others as well. Last October 23, 2008, the New York University Medical Center launched the Support Group Meeting for its Limb Loss Rehabilitation Program. It was an open forum. My mom introduced me to the audience which consisted of six former NYUMC amputee patients and their families, two prosthetists (one of them an amputee himself), some medical residents, nurses, and other NYU Medical Center staff. I spoke about my experience, continuing struggles, and accomplishments.

> *Life has been hard; but life has also been kind.*

On December 18, 2008, our NYU support group meeting was televised by a local channel where I was interviewed together with other quadruple amputees. I felt so privileged to be part of the group that I would like to take it a step

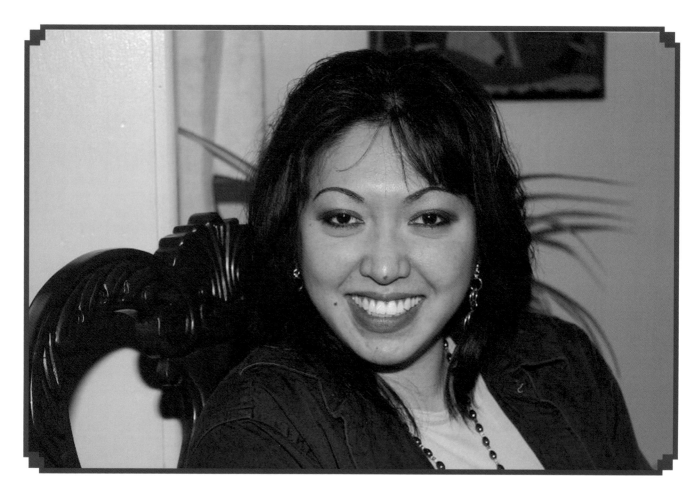

Sheila May A. Advento lives and works in New Jersey.

further. I am registered to attend a peer counselor training program and will try to get certified so I can provide support to my fellow amputees. I hope that sharing my story can be a source of comfort to them and their families.

I believe in the power of the human spirit to survive. It is up to us to persist and turn our losses into gifts.

~ Sheila May A. Advento, Hackensack, NJ

"*It is up to us to persist and turn our losses into gifts.*"

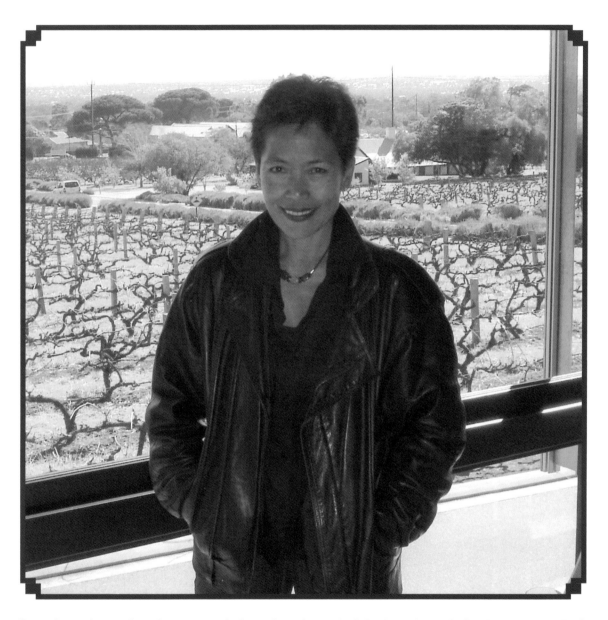

Cynthia Angeles lives with her husband, Michael, in Washington, DC.

Acknowledgments

This book would not have been possible without the help of my family. They are all part of this in spirit. I would like to thank my aunt, Cynthia Angeles, for helping me write and develop this book, and to Michael Nowak, her husband, for his valuable input and support of this project. We owe special thanks to Michael Lesparre for his advice and patience to read through all our drafts; and to my cousin, Ophelia (Piah) Panganiban, for her comments and help in editing the manuscript.

The photos were taken by various friends and family members; the book cover is based on my portrait, an oil painting by my aunt, Cynthia Angeles.

A Funny Thing

A new path with open eyes

Destined for completeness

Capturing old flames

As souls grow with each day of the sun's rays.

Blessed with tranquility,

Blessed with strength,

And keeping oneself

Builds the foundation of what may seem like

A Dream.

Thoughts of such face and memories lingered

And now here...

The birth of an overwhelming clarity

Brings forth nothing more but great

Possibilities

And yet keeping what is present

And aware of any challenges.

This intense feeling is somewhat

A Funny Thing.

~ Sheila May A. Advento

LaVergne, TN USA
30 September 2009
159418LV00001BA